AF322908

THE JOYS—AND DANGERS—OF CONTACT LENSES

by

Jack Hartstein, M.D.

A Hearthstone Book

Carlton Press, Inc.   New York, N.Y.

CONTENTS

FOREWORD

Contact lenses are becoming an increasingly popular modality for correcting various types of visual defects. Lenses currently available include daily and extended wear soft contact lenses, oxygen or gas permeable lenses of various designs, and lenses to alter eye color.

But...all the news isn't good! The Center for Disease Control (CDC) in Atlanta reports an increasing number of documented cases of Acanthamoeba Keratitis. This devastating parasitic infection can cause the loss of an eye. In *The Joys—And Dangers—Of Contact Lenses,* Dr. Jack Hartstein lists recommendations for the prevention of this ravaging disease. Bacterial and viral infections, infections by fungi, protozoa and a myriad of other contact lens related problems are addressed in this slim volume written in non-technical terms.

The Joys—And Dangers—Of Contact Lenses is the first book of this kind written in a patient/doctor case history format. This easy read is a must for the 22 million contact lens wearers and those considering being fitted with contact lenses in the future.

THE JOYS—AND DANGERS—OF CONTACT LENSES

Dorothy Parker was right! At least 22 million contact lens wearers think so. This increasingly popular aid for correcting vision generates a myriad of questions, a number of caveats and a need for precise information.

In recognizing danger signals, the patient is guided all along the way with vignettes that illustrate virtually every facet and fact that may arise with the care and use of contact lenses. This book lifts the veil of mystery to enlighten in an entertaining format. Caveats also include information on individuals who are poor contact lens candidates and the effects of cosmetics on contact lenses. The result is a population made confident, well informed and alerted to the dangers resulting from contacts and their prevention, leading to a healthier life style.

Credentials:

Associate Professor, Clinical Ophthalmology, Washington University, St. Louis, Missouri. Director, Contact Lens Clinics, Barnes Hospital, St. Louis, Missouri.

Published Works:

Questions and Answers on Contact Lenses, 1968
Extend Wear Lenses in Myopia and Aphakia, 1982
Editor, *Contact and Intraocular Lens Medical Journal,* 1973, 1983.

THE JOYS—AND DANGERS— OF CONTACT LENSES

1
DANGERS FROM HOT TUBS

"Don't anybody move!" shouted Susan. "Fred just lost his contact lens!" The five others in the hot tub stopped splashing.

"How did you lose your lens?"

"I don't know, Maria. I just rubbed my eye and it fell out. That doesn't happen very often."

"Let's all be still," Diane suggested. "Let the water settle and maybe we can see it at the bottom of the tub."

"I think I see it," Archie said, "down there toward the middle at the bottom."

You don't wear contacts, Archie. Why don't you try to get it?"

"O.K., Alice. Everybody stay perfectly still now, don't make any waves. I have it. Here you go, Fred. Boy, it sure is a flimsy thing."

"You got that right. Thanks, Arch. In fact, it's so thin, sometimes I can't tell when it's inside out, but these contacts sure are comfortable. I've left them in my eyes for over two months without taking them out."

"Say, Fred, do you have to clean it up or something before you put it back in your eye?"

"Oh, no, it's been in water and I'm sure it's all right," Fred replied, and slipped the contact lens in place.

Several months passed. Fred was sitting in English class.

"What's the matter, Fred? You contact lenses bothering you?"

"Sort of, Janet. My eyes are itching. Guess my allergies are flaring up again."

"You don't think it has anything to do with that time you lost your lens in the hot tub, do you?" Janet asked.

"No, that has nothing to do with it. I've lost a lens before and nothing like this ever happened."

"Why don't you go see your eye doctor?" said Janet.

"I think I will," replied Fred. "Last time he gave me some cortisone eye drops for my allergies and it helped a lot. Maybe I can give him a call; he might send me some without even seeing me. I really don't know if I have time to go to his office."

The next day Janet met Fred as they were entering English class. He was rubbing his eyes even more vigorously. "Did you call the eye doctor?"

"Sure I did, but he wouldn't send me the drops without seeing me. I have an appointment to see him the day after tomorrow at 2:00 o'clock."

"Good. Let me know what happens. Your left eye especially looks irritated."

Two days later, Fred was sitting in the examination chair in Dr. Michaels' office.

"Good to see you, Fred," the doctor said, looking at his patient's chart. "Fred, you haven't been here in two years. Haven't you received our reminders? I told you that with extended wear contact lenses, you had to return for periodic follow-up visits."

"I meant to, Dr. Michaels, but I have been so busy...but here I am, and from now on I promise to keep my appointments."

"What symptoms are you having?" inquired Dr. Michaels.

"Well, my eyes itch and they burn and ache. They hurt at times, and quite often when I wake up in the morning, they're stuck together so tight I can hardly get them open."

"Have you been wearing your contact lenses the entire time?"

"Yes, I've become so dependent on them, that I don't even know where my glasses are."

"How often do you take them out to clean them?"

"Oh, I suppose every four to eight weeks. Sometimes even longer, if they are not bothering me."

"Well, let's take a look. Place your chin on the chin rest in this slit lamp. It's used as a microscope to examine your eyes under magnification."

"What do you see?"

"Now, don't get worried," soothed Dr. Michaels. "This is just an examination. I'll let you know what I find, and then we'll discuss it." Dr. Michaels then proceeded to carefully examine

Fred's eye with varying degrees of magnification, looking at all the layers of the eye carefully. "Ah!" he exclaimed. "Fred, you have developed a little ulceration here, with a tiny bit of loose tissue on top. I have my suspicions so I'm going to take a little sample of some of these cells, and send them to the laboratory to make a proper diagnosis. You can sit back now, Fred. In the meantime, I'll give you a mild cortisone preparation. It should alleviate your symptoms of itching and burning. We'll make an appointment for you to return in three days, then I'll be able to tell if you're responding to the treatment. The laboratory results will be back by then, and I'll have a better idea of your problem."

Three days later, Fred was again seated in Dr. Michaels' office.

"How are your eyes feeling this morning?" inquired Dr. Michaels.

"Oh, much, much better," replied Fred. "Those drops you prescribed were wonderful! I guess it was an allergy after all."

"Not quite," said Dr. Michaels. "I wish it were that easy. I'm afraid I have bad news for you."

"What do you mean, bad news?" asked Fred, a note of concern creeping into his voice.

"Well, you remember that little sample I took of your eye and sent to the laboratory? They tested it for a special type of infection and the news isn't good."

"What type of infection?" asked Fred.

"The diagnosis came back Amoebic Keratitis. That's an inflammation of the cornea, due to amoeba."

"Amoeba Keratitis? What is that?"

"Well, Fred, I think we better go over this very carefully, because I want you to understand what we are up against."

Fred became more anxious than ever.

"Well," Dr. Michaels replied, "I don't want to worry you unduly, but we're in for a long and arduous course of treatment, so it's important for you to understand the seriousness of your condition. I need your full cooperation."

"You have it, you have it. Just tell me what do I have, what's wrong with me?"

"Well, let's begin at the beginning," answered Dr. Michaels. "You may recall from you biology days that an amoeba is a single celled animal, which occurs either singly or in a colony formation.

It belongs to the family of Protozoa. These are minute unicellular animals capable of carrying on all life processes. There are many in the family of protozoa and relatively few actually attack men; still fewer are associated with pathology."

"Pardon me for interrupting you, Dr. Michaels," said Fred, "but I now recall from my biology days that there is a disease called Amoebic Dysentery caused by one type of amoeba. I believe it was called Endamoeba Histolytica."

"You're right, Fred. Actually, that organism was first discovered in 1875. It is estimated that approximately ten percent of the world's population harbors that parasite. But what we're talking about has nothing to do with dysentery. This type of amoeba causes an inflammation of the cornea called Keratitis, and I'm afraid that we ophthalmologists have been misdiagnosing or missing it altogether, because the incidence has been relatively rare. In fact, as far as I can tell, there are only about a hundred cases that have been diagnosed in the United States. Amoeba are present all over the world. They've been found in fresh water, well water, soil, barley, and even in the air in London. They've been found in hot tubs, too."

"Hot tubs!" exclaimed Fred.

"Hot tubs. Why are you so excited about hot tubs?"

"Well, I like hot tubs and I've been in a few recently. A couple of months ago I lost one of my contact lenses while I was in a hot tub. I thought I was pretty lucky to find it."

"What did you do when you found it?"

"Well, I put it right back in my eye."

"Did you wash it off?"

"No, it was in the water, so I assumed it was clean."

"Well, it is quite possible that could have been the source of this infection. Fred, this is really a strange organism. It exists in nature in two forms: as a trophozoite, that is, a little animal that moves around, and also a double walled cyst. That means in adverse conditions, for example, when it gets cold or dry, this animal can turn into a round ball with a hard outer coating. This allows it to survive under these circumstances. In 1958 several investigators demonstrated that free living amoeba can cause brain lesions in mice and monkeys, and they theorize that it also can cause disease in humans. Following their reports, the first human infection by free living amoeba was reported in 1965. It was found in an Australian man who died of meningitis. There is another reason I want to to come in to have your contact lenses inspected on a regular basis. Soft contact lenses gather deposits— that little crust you see on the lenses. Those deposits, which sometimes are calcium or other protein deposits, collect bacteria— a particular type of bacteria. It's been found these little amoeba animals flourish by eating the bacteria. Therefore, you see that if you have dirty lenses with deposits, they collect bacteria which attracts amoeba."

"But, Dr. Michaels, how does it get from the lens into my eye?"

"It stands to reason that when a person wears a contact lens, he probably sustains very minor abrasions or breaks in the epithelium, a thin transparent front surface of the cornea. Any injury to the cornea or any break in the tissue can be a means of the amoeba gaining entrance to the eye."

"How can I tell if I have this infection without going to the eye doctor?" asked Fred.

"Even opthalmologists have a difficult time with this disease. In the beginning, one might see just some tiny little ulcers, or an iritis might develop."

"What's iritis?" Fred asked.

"It's a soreness or achiness due to inflammation of the iris. It causes a patient to be very sensitive to light."

"That's me," said Fred. "I just can't stand the light."

"The inflammation then continues slowly, until there is a ringed shaped infiltrate—a ring forming on the clear cornea. By that time the diagnosis can easily be made. Eye pain is often very severe. Many Ophthalmologists may at first confuse this with herpes infections of the eye."

"Well, how can you be sure what it is?"

"With a laboratory diagnosis. There's a chemofluorescent called Calcofluor White which attaches to part of the amoebic cyst called the Polysaccharide Polymer. This calcofluor can also reliably detect fungus infections in scrapings of the cornea, and it's a simple, quick and highly reliable test that diagnosis Acanthamoeba Keratitis."

"Gee whiz!" exclaimed Fred, "what should I do now? You can clear this up, can't you?"

Patiently Dr. Michaels continued.

"I hate to say this, Fred, but the preferred treatment of acanthamoeba keratitis has not been determined. Various laboratory tests have demonstrated that the trophozoite—that's the living, active form of the amoeba—can be killed by a variety of antibiotic agents, but the cysts are highly resistant. A variety of drugs offer some hope, but in a number of cases a cornea transplant might be necessary to remove the disease from your eye. Fortunately, many eyes like yours have been saved through the various available treatments."

"Doctor, how can I avoid this type of infection?"

"We don't know all the answers, but the following rules should be observed:

1. The inability of normal levels of chlorine in swimming pools to eliminate acanthamoeba cysts has been documented. Therefore, one should not routinely wear contact lenses in hot tubs or when swimming.

2. Do not make your own saline using distilled or tap water with salt tablets.

3. When using bottled unpreserved saline, do not use the large, multi-containers because the solution can become contaminated. Use smaller, disposable, one-time containers.

4. Always wash your hands before touching your contact lenses. This is a must, because there are probably many more of these amoebic organisms on your hands than in the water.

5. Whenever possible, use heat disinfection for your soft contact lenses, even if they're extended wear. Chemical disinfection, that is the solutions on the market called 'cold sterilization,' do not destroy the cysts as far as we know.

6. Most important, should a person develop eye pain, reduced vision, discharge from the yes, or redness, he should immediately be seen by an ophthalmologist.

"I see now how negligent I've been, Dr. Michaels. Believe me, I'll take all the precautions in the future. And thanks for the information and your help."

2

YOUR EYES ARE WARPED

"Tim, where'd I put my contact lenses?" Nancy groped around the bedroom.

"I don't know. Don't you always put them in the same place?"

"Yes, I usually leave them on the dresser. I drank a little too much at that party last night, and I got in so late, I don't know where I put them."

"Well, why don't you put on your glasses and wear them until we find your contact lenses?"

"I can't see through the glasses. I never could see through them after I got the contact lenses."

"Then why did we spend all that money on glasses if you can't see through them?"

"I don't know, I don't know. Please! Help me find my contact lenses. I can't go to work unless I find them," Nancy cried.

"I have no idea where they are," Tim said. "I guess I'll have to lead you by the hand, and take you to work in my car."

"Don't be silly, Tim. I can't work if I can't see."

"What do you want me to do?" exclaimed Tim, becoming exasperated. "It's early in the morning and here we are having an argument already! I know! I'll call Dr. Rafferty when the office opens and see if I can get an emergency appointment," Tim offered. "Then we'll find out what is going on. Maybe he has a spare pair of contact lenses in his office that you can use until we order you a second pair. We may even be able to find these."

"I sure wish I knew where I put them," Nancy whined, as she

17

continued searching. It was useless. They were nowhere to be found. Nancy put on her glasses reluctantly. Everything was blurred and distorted, but she had to wear something. Tim just couldn't understand why she was unable to see through her glasses. "What's the use of wearing glasses if you can't see through them?" he asked.

"Well, it's better than nothing," said Nancy. "I can see a little!" Glumly, she sighed.

Promptly at eight, Tim called Dr. Rafferty's office. "Please let me talk to him," Tim said. "This is an emergency."

"Come right over," Dr. Rafferty advised after hearing the story. "We'll work you in."

At eight-thirty they were at Dr. Rafferty's office, and ten minutes later were in his treatment room.

"Tell me what happened," the doctor said.

"I've lost my contact lenses. I have no idea where they are. I know I should have a spare pair, but I don't. And, Doctor, I'm blind, I need the lenses badly."

"Why can't she see through her glasses when she takes off the contact lenses, doctor?"

"My records show you haven't been back here for over six years. Let's see what has happened in the meantime. Lean forward and place your head in this instrument so I can see and measure your corneas."

"What is that instrument, Dr. Rafferty?" Nancy asked.

"It's a Keratometer, an instrument for measuring the curvature of your eye on which the contact lenses rest." Dr. Rafferty examined the surface of the corneas and studied the various meridians or directions. "You have developed quite an astigmatism, Nancy."

"Astigmatism? What's that?"

"Well, let's say that your eyes have become warped."

"That sounds terrible," Nancy and Tim said in unison. "When something is warped, it sounds like it needs straightening. Can her eyes be straightened out?"

"I believe they can, Tim. Well," explained Dr. Rafferty, "the condition goes back a long ways. In the mid-1960s, a major problem associated with long term wearing of hard contact lenses was reported: high amounts of With The Rule astigmatism were found, as much as six dioters following lens removal. That means that the corneas were warped in a vertical direction. Future studies confirmed that finding. In fact, many lens wearers develop increases in this warping several days after lenses are removed. Since the eye no longer has its round shape, determining the prescription for a pair of glasses is a difficult task. The warping, or the astigmatism, may change from week to week. As you know, many people have worn contact lenses now for twenty or more years and neglected visits to their eye doctor. As I said, you haven't been back here in a six years. We have found that in most cases that after about three or four weeks without contact lenses the curvature of the eye may stabilize, and at that time a patient can be refitted with contact lenses or tested for glasses."

"Three or four week!" exclaimed Nancy. "I'll be fired. I need to see right now!"

"I know, I know," replied Dr. Rafferty. "You're a lucky young woman. We can do something that will help. In the past, doctors urged patients to go without their lenses and checked them every couple of weeks until the curvature of the eye quit changing. Another method was to fit such a person with soft contact lenses, which though not restoring perfect vision, would give back some of the vision until the eyes quit changing. But now we have a new type of contact lens, a lens that breathes oxygen. It's a Gas Permeable Contact Lens. I will make up a pair of these lenses based on the same curve as the ones you lost. Fortunately, for most people the curvature of the eyes returns to normal with this type of oxygen breathing contact lens. But let this be a warning to you, Nancy. Don't stay away so long!"

3

"MY EYE IS KILLING ME"

"My eyes are killing me," Charles complained to his roommate Henry. "I can't even open them."

"Come on, Charles, we're late for class."

"Just go on without me," said Charles.

"No. I can't leave you alone. Get in the car and I'll take you over to the hospital emergency room. It is just across the campus and the doctor can take a look."

"O.K., Henry. I sure appreciate it. I really feel terrible."

Henry helped Charles get in the car. He drove across the campus and soon Charles was sitting in the doctor's office. The emergency room doctor, a young man who also wore contact lenses, was sympathetic to Charles' plight. He instilled a drop of anesthetic in each eye, and after a couple minutes, Charles opened his eyes and said, "Wow! I can see again. Thanks a lot, Doc. Well, I am ready to go. You've cured me."

"Not quite," came the reply. "Let me look at you with the slit lamp, the magnifying microscope." The doctor noticed a cloudy spot on his patient's left eye. "You better wait here. I am going to call the ophthalmologist on duty to come and see you."

"I sure hate to miss class. Can't I go and come back this afternoon? My eyes feel fine now."

"The only reason they feel fine," explained the emergency room eye doctor, "is because I've numbed your eyes, but it's only temporary. In five or ten minutes, you'll be in excruciating pain again. Just wait here. You can always take another class, but you can't get another pair of eyes."

"That's true, young man. I'm Dr. Hartlain. What's this I hear

20

about your eyes?"

"Well, I was fine last night, but this morning when I woke up I couldn't open my eyes, and the pain was terrible. But I feel fine now."

"That's because the emergency room physician instilled an anesthetic in your eye. It's only temporary and you're not cured, but it does make it more comfortable for you and allows us to examine your eyes. My goodness, that is quite an ulcer you have."

"Ulcer!" exclaimed Charles. "What's that?"

"Well," explained Dr. Hartlain, "it's a very serious infection that's involved the tissues of the cornea or the front window of your eye. It's like an acid that's eaten through part of your eye."

"Acid?"

"No, not exactly acid, but a certain type of bacteria. I could start treatment by prescribing a broad spectrum antibiotic."

"What's a broad spectrum antibiotic?"

"It's a combination of antibiotics that will attack most infections, but I do believe the safer course for us to follow is to obtain a culture. I'll take a sample of the infection on a sterile cotton swab, send it to the bacteriology laboratory, where it will be tested and the germ that's causing the infection will be identified. I'm also going to ask them to find out its sensitivities."

"You've lost me now."

"This enables us to determine which antibiotics are effective against that particular germ. First, a germ is placed on a special nutrient, where it multiplies rapidly. When the plate is covered with that particular germ, a little of the antibiotic is placed all over this plate and wherever a clear area occurs, we know that the antibiotic is effective."

"Gee, that is fascinating," replied Charles.

"We can do something else right now," said Dr. Hartlain. "One of these swabs is going to be spread across a slide and then, with the use of certain chemicals, we'll have a good idea what type of germ it is."

"What do you mean, what type of germ it is?" asked Charles.

"This idea was developed by Dr. Gram, who discovered that by taking a certain blue dye and covering the slide with it, then washing it off, the blue dye was absorbed by certain germs. These are called Gram Positive. Not all germs absorbed the blue color, so he spread a red color over the glass plate, washed that off, and those germs that absorbed the red color were called Gram Negative,"

"But why is it important to know if something is Gram positive or Gran negative?"

"Well, we have found that certain antibiotics, like penicillin, are effective against blue germs, the Gram positive germs. Other antibiotics, such as streptomycin or neomycin, are effective against the red germs, or Gram negative germs."

"Wow! That's really fascinating," Charles exclaimed. "What do germs look like, Dr. Hartlain?" questioned Charles.

"Let's take a look." Dr. Hartlain took a sample of the secretion from charles' eye, smeared some on a tiny glass plate, and went through the Gram stain procedure, first using blue dye, washing it off, then using red dye, again washing it off. He placed the slide under a microscope. "Take a look, Charles. What do you see?"

"Well, I see little rod-like structures."

What color are they?"

"Kind of red," he answered. As he looked up from the microscope, he saw concern creep across Dr. Hartlain's face.

"Well, son, we do have a very serious infection on our hands. It most likely is a germ we call Pseudomonas Aeruginosa. What kind of contact lenses do you have?"

"Oh, I wear Extended Wear Contact Lenses," Charles replied. "I've worn them for six years without any problem. In fact, I have had no trouble at all until this morning."

"How do you sterilize them?"

"I use any one of the preparations from the drug store, whichever one's the cheapest. I try to cut costs wherever I can. But what is this about pseudomonas, Dr. Hartlain?"

"Well, Charles, recent studies indicate that pseudomonas infection is quite common in extended wear contact lens patients. Some investigators feel that this is related to the deposits that collect on this type of lens. The deposits attract this pseudomonas bacteria, and once there is an overwhelming amount of this bacteria on the lens, it only takes a scratch on the eye to afford an entrance site for the germ to enter the cornea. Interestingly enough, it has been found that most corneal ulcers caused by bacteria in patients who don't wear contact lenses are caused by a Gram positive organism called the Staphylococcus. This is a round organism that takes a blue stain or Gram positive. This is quite different from the ulcer you have. Charles, this is one of the most feared bacteria in opthalmology. We worry about this very same germ during eye surgery, because an eye can be lost within twenty-four hours after being attacked by pseudomonas. Fortunately for you, because we diagnosed the problem early, there is an excellent chance of saving your eye."

"Please do all you can, Doctor."

"I will. But you must learn to follow the instruction that were delivered along with your contact lenses."

4

"ACHOO!"

"Are your allergies acting up again, Ellen?"

"I'll say, Dale. I can hardly go outside. My eyes just itch, and worst of all, I'm having a hard time wearing my contact lenses."

"So wear your glasses during the hayfever season."

"You know how I hate to be seen in glasses, but I guess I'll have to unless I can find some way to get through this allergy season."

"Have you asked you ophthalmologist if there is anything he can do to keep you in contact lenses during this period?"

"Oh, I've just been too busy to see him, but I just can't put up with this terrible itching anymore."

"I'll call Dr. Mountbil right now and see if he can work you in today. I know he likes to see his contact lens patients immediately, especially if they're having a problem." Ellen dabbed at her eyes with a tissue as Dale dialed the doctor's office. "Dr. Mountbil can't see you until 3:00 this afternoon, so I'll go on to work. Why don't you just keep that appointment and I'll pick you up after work."

"I can see what the trouble is already," said Dr. Mountbil, "but I'll aske you anyway, young lady. Tell me how your eyes bother you."

"Well, during this hayfever seasoon I can hardly keep my eyes open, they itch so badly that I want to rub then all the time, and they water constantly. I've tried a number of eye drops that claim they're good for itchy eyes, but nothing seems to help. I want to keep wearing my contact lenses but it sure is a problem. I hate the idea of wearing glasses!"

"Well, first let's have a look," said Dr. Mountbil as he examine her eyes with various instruments. Part of the examination included everting her upper eyelid by turning the upper eyelid inside out so the doctor can see if there are little bumps under the upper eyelid. Ellen was asked to look to the right, left, up and down. The interior of her eye was examined, eye pressure was taken, and her eyes examined with a slit lamp (all the normal things that an ophthalmologist does).

"Allergic conjunctivitis!" Dr. Mountbil declared.

"I could have told you that, but what do I do about if?"

"Well, since your eye pressure is normal and there are no breaks in the corneal epithelium, we can safely give you a steroid eye drop like cortizone for a short period of time. It will relieve the itching. There is a recent preparation which will keep alleviating your symptoms."

"What's that?"

"It's called Chromolyn, and was developed in England. It's administered in a four percent solution and we'll prescribe two drops to be used four to six times a day for at least two months."

"How does it work?" Ellen, a registered nurse, was always interested in new medications.

"There is a type of cell called a mast cell," Dr. Mountbil began, "and it is estimated there are about fifty thousand of these cells in the fluids and tissues surrounding each eye. These mast cells contain histamine, a type of chemical. When this mast cell is attacked by an allergic stimulus, the histamine pours out and causes a severe intense itching. Chromolyn prevents the mast cell from rupturing. Actually, Ellen, it's quite complicated. It appears that the stimulus that causes the mast cell to break causes calcium to enter the cell and Chromolyn prevents calcium from entering the cell, so since the cell does not receive the calcium, it does not break open and release its histamine. You will have to use this medication for at least two to three weeks before you'll begin to feel any benefit. You probably will have to use it during the entire allergy season. The cortizone eye drop will give you immediate relief and carry you until the Chromolyn preparation can take over. What you have is not serious, so don't worry. But I'm sure it is terribly aggravating and prevents you from wearing your contact lenses comfortably."

"Why did you turn my upper eyelids inside out, Dr. Mount-bil?"

"Well, I was looking for another condition called Giant Papillary Conjunctivitis, or abbreviated GPC."

"What is GPC?" inquired Ellen. "Sure sounds terrible!"

"Well, it's not life threatening, but it certainly can be an aggravating problem for both the ophthalmologist and the patient. Some people theorize that the contact lens, and particularly soft contact lenses, absorb certain chemicals from tears which then act as an antigen or exciting agent to the under surface of the eyelid, causing an allergic type of reaction. When an opthalmologist turns the upper lid inside out, he looks for characteristic bumps called papillae, which tells him the degree of GPC that is present."

"Can GPC be treated?" asked Ellen.

"Yes," replied Dr. Mountbil, "but it's quite difficult. First of all, one needs to remove the contact lenses. Some ophthalmologists advise removing the contact lenses totally for a period of two to four weeks while treating this condition with a combination of cortizone and opticrome. Other ophthalmologists switch their patients to different brands of contact lenses while they're undergoing treatment and still other doctors switch patients to hard lenses or oxygen permeable contact lenses which are made of a rigid material. The combination of medications and the switch to different types of lenses hopefully result in a cure, or at least a control, for many suffering patients with Giant Papillary conjunctivitis."

"Well, I'm certainly glad I don't have GPC, Dr. Mountbil. It sounds like a long drawn out recovery time."

"It is indeed. Be sure to follow my instructions and don't forget regular check-ups, Ellen."

"For sure, Dr. Mountbil, and thanks."

5

"I SEE RED"

"What's the problem, Ralph? Why are you always looking at me like that?"

"Well, you're a beautiful girl, Debbie, but whenever I look at you, I see red."

"What's that supposed to mean?"

"I mean that when I look at you I see red eyes. Why don't you quit wearing those contact lenses?"

"You know I can't see without them, Ralph. So why do you keep pestering me?"

"Don't you see yourself?" Surely you look in the mirror. Do you like seeing those red eyes?"

"No, I don't...besides, they itch, but what else can I do?"

"You could wear glasses."

"Ugh! I don't want to wear glasses."

"Then why don't you find out why your eyes are red."

"Maybe I should."

"When is the last time you saw Dr. Rogin?"

"It's been at least two years. I just don't have the money to pay for those office visits. You know he's awfully high."

"Well, darn it, Debbie, make an appointment. I'll pay for this visit."

"My, my, young lady, you certainly do have a problem," Dr. Rogin said, scrutinizing his patient.

"That's why I'm here. Ralph thinks so, too," Debbie replied, avoiding his eyes.

"Well, let's first begin by giving you a thorough eye exam.

You haven't been here in over two years and we have to rule out any underlying disease processes."

"You mean I have a disease?"

"No, we just have to make sure."

"Can contact lenses cause a disease?" questioned Debbie.

"Of course they can. Automobiles can cause accidents, but that doesn't mean that one should quit driving. It's just necessary to observe a certain degree of prudence!" Dr. Rogin proceeded to throughly examine Debbie's eyes, cheking her vision with and without her contact lenses, measuring her refraction, which results in a prescription that will give her satisfactory vision. He examined and measured the cornea, the front surface of the eye, with the keratometer, which measures the curvatures of the eye, and a slit lamp that measures the health of the tissues of the eye. He then checked her retinal circulation, the health of the optic nerve, and ruled out any conditions that might disturb the interior of the eye. After satisfying himself that her eyes were perfectly normal and free of infection, Dr. Rogin questioned Debbie about her contact solutions.

"Do you have the solution you use to wet the contact lenses and the one you use to store your contact lenses?"

"Yes, I have them right here in my purse," Debbie replied, reaching for the two bottles.

"Hmmm," thought Dr. Rogin, as he read the ingredients on both bottles. "I see that they both contain Thimerosol."

"What's that?" asked Debbie. "Sounds pretty heavy."

"No, no," replied Dr. Rogin, "it's merely one of the chemicals in your solution. Actually, it's the chemical that disinfects your contact lenses."

"So what's the problem with thimerosol?" Debbie was puzzled.

"Thimerosol is a mercurochrome containing compound and dermatologists report that at least fifty percent of the population is sensitive to mercurochrome products. It could well be that your entire problem is due to a sensitibity to this particular chemical."

"I didn't think a chemical or solution that was supposed to sterilize and purify my contact lenses could cause my eyes to be red."

"It's a trade-off," replied Dr. Rogin. "It is effective in sterilizing your contact lenses, but we find that approximately twenty percent of the patients can't tolerate that solution."

"Why not?" asked Debbie.

"Well, it often causes reactions, red eyes and sensitivity, just like you're showing. All we need you to do," Dr. Rogin said, "is to change your solutions and make sure that none of the solutions you'll be using contain thimerosol. Because thimerosol is such an effective agent, Debbie, I want you to check every eye drop and eye wash to make sure they are not preserving it with thimerosol. Many antibiotic eye drops, artificial tear drops—in fact, all kinds of eye drops—contain thimerosol. So to play it safe, look at all the ingredients of any drop you'll be putting in your eyes to be sure it does not contain thimerosol. Solutions I have been switching some of my patients to are those containing hydrogen peroxide."

"Hydrogen peroxide," exclaimed Debbie. "Isn't that the same thing people use to bleach their hair or swish out their mouths.?"

"That's the one," replied Dr. Rogin. "Three percent hydrogen peroxide is a very effective sterilizing solution and a number of types of peroxide systems are presently on the market. On the one hand, there is heat sterilization for certain types of contact lenses, but for those using chemical sterilization, most eye doctors have come to the conclusion that hydrogen peroxide is the treatment of choice."

"Thank you, Dr. Rogin." Debbie sighed with relief. "I'll follow your advice and hope my red eyes disappear."

"I'm sure you'll be fine. Just don't forget to report any discomfort or discharge from eyes. And don't forget to read and check every label."

"You bet I will," Debbie smiled.

6

"NOTHING IS FOREVER"

"How long have you worn these contact lenses, Anne?" Dr. Klinelord asked during the examination of his patient as he was examining her eyes.

"Well, I guess these lenses are at least two years old, but they never give me any trouble. It's just that I don't see too well any more."

"Didn't I advise you, Anne, that once you received these extended wear lenses, you were to come back every four to six months for follow-up visits? Extended wear means you don't have to remove them every evening. It doesn't mean extended time between visits for eye exams."

"I know, Dr. Klinelord, but I've been away at college, and the time got away from me."

"Surely there are eye doctors in Boston."

"Yes, but they're all busy and the college is thirteen miles from town, and it's just too much effort."

"Well, you certainly are a lucky young lady so far. Fortunately your eyes are particularly healthy and my examination shows no pathology whatsoever. But your lenses are terribly smudged and dirty."

"What happens when a lens gets old, Dr. Klinelord?"

"From the day a soft lens is placed in your eye, it starts to age, Anne. It gradually loses its water content and becomes more and more like a rigid lens. that is, it becomes steeper and starts to get layered with deposits. Several investigators have shown that layered deposits form within the first four to six hours that contact lenses are worn. It's not all bad news, though. More often

30

than not, those people who develop infections don't do so until the lenses are considerably older. My personal opinion is that even the most successful wearers should replace their lenses every year. For safety's sake and for the health of the eyes, a patient should obtain new lenses every six months. My daughter has worn the same prescription for over eight years and I send her a pair every four to six months. I am happy to tell you her eyes have remained completely healthy in all respects, with no signs of any disease whatsoever."

"Well," replied Anne, "that's all well and good for your daughter because you can send her the lenses and not charge her. These lenses are quite expensive and I can't afford new ones every four to six months, nor can many of my friends."

"Anne," replied Dr. Klinelord, "you've targeted the problem manufacturers and eye doctors all over the country are addressing. We know it's important to reduce the costs of lenses, especially to soft lens clients. Some ideas we're spearheading include warranties or insurance policies from manufacturers, and ways and means of cutting manufacturing costs. People must have an opportunity to obtain new lenses every four to six months, at reasonable costs. This is the best way to avoid complications from contact lenses. The newer Oxygen Permeable Hard Contact lenses don't need replacing as often. However, studies are beginning to indicate that even those lenses need to be discarded and exchanged every eighteen months to two years, because the deposits they develop could be injurious to the eye."

"But what about my vision, Dr. Klinelord. I think I need stronger contact lenses."

"Anne," replied Dr. Klinelord, "your examination shows that your vision has remained essentially the same. You will see that when we replace these worn lenses with new lenses of the same prescription. Your vision will be up to 20/20."

"Thank you, Dr. Klinelord," replied Anne. "I am certainly happy to learn my eyes are O.K. See you in six months—and that's a promise."

"THERE ARE FRENCHMEN AND FRENCHMEN"

"Let me tell you a story," Dr. Pierre addressed the medical student. "It will then help me explain to you the kind of corneal ulcer you have."

"As you know, I am of French extraction. I was invited to a heavy-weight prize fight, something I have never witnessed. By the eighth round, one of the fighters was being horribly beaten. His nose appeared broken, blood was running from his mouth, he was knocked to the canvas, and the referee was starting to count him out, when someone said, "Get up, Frenchy, get up, Frenchy." I couldn't stand it any longer. I immediately leaped from my seat and made a mad dash toward the ring. I don't know where I found the strength, but I climbed through the ropes and, catching the other fighter by surprise, I bounced him sharply on the ear. He turned around as if a wasp or mosquito had stung him, and started to come at me, when the referee came between us. One of the referees recognized me and exclaimed, "Dr. Pierre, what are you doing in the prize ring?"

"I don't know myself," I exclaimed, "but a Frenchman was knocked to the canvas. I couldn't sit idly by."

"Oh, Dr. Pierre," replied the referee, "you are wrong. He is not French, that is just his name—Frenchy."

"That taught me a lesson. Things aren't always the way they appear. The ulcer you show is an ulcer without bacteria, as opposed to an ulcer with germs. You have what is called a Marginal Corneal Ulcer."

"What is a marginal corneal ulcer, Dr. Pierre?"

"Well, picture the eye, the cornea, like the windshield of your

eye, except that it's round, and near the edge there is a clear
border. Within that border, there are a few little white dots.
These are called Marginal Corneal Ulcers. We don't find bacteria
in these ulcers, but I will take a culture or a sample of the
secretions on your eyelashes and eyelids, and we'll see just what
kind of infection you have."

"My eyes have always been red," Sandford explained. "When
I was a kid they said I had 'granulated eyelids,' whatever that
means."

"In any case, you cannot wear your contact lenses while this
conditions is going on. This condition is called Blepharocon-
junctivitis, or chronic eyelid infection, and should have been
cleared up before you were placed in contact lenses."

Dr. Pierre then took a sample of secretion and spread it on a
slide and went through the procedure of the Gram stain. First,
he poured blue dye over the slide, washing it off with a neutraliz-
ing solution, then pouring red dye and washing it off. He asked
Sanford to come look through the microscope. Sanford was a
medical student and eager to understand this study. Through
the microscope, Sanford observed little round cicles stained blue,
meaning Gram positive, and some stained red, meaning negative.
Dr. Pierre explained the little round circles are called cocci.

"So," Dr. Pierre said to Sanford, "at least we know that you
have a coccus infection and now we're going to plate it out on a
medium which allows bacteria to grow. If it grows in clumps or
colonies, it is streptococcus."

Two days later Dr. Pierre showed Sanford a glass plate, containing the nutrient Agar. What Sanford witnessed were clumps of
yellow colonies. These golden, yellow colonies are Staphylococcus,
Dr. Pierre explained.

"You have a staph infection of the eyelids. It can be treated
by scrubbing your eyelids and getting rid of all the scales. You'll
also need an antibiotic ointment. After we clear up the condition
you can resume wearing your contact lenses. I'll prescribe a mild
cortizone eye drop, too. This will help with the allergic reaction
you have toward this staph. You don't have infected ulcers. As
I explained in the beginning, there are Frenchmen and there are
Frenchmen."

"Thank you, Dr. Pierre. I was frightened by that word, ulcer."

NOT ALL CONES ARE ASSOCIATED WITH ICE CREAM

This is a true story. Three years ago, I received a letter from my cousin in London, informing me of a peculiar eye condition affecting his grandson. He stated that Doron had been to three different eye specialists through the British Eye Health Service, and though they reported no infections or diseases of the retina or the eye, this child's best corrected vision was 20/200, or 20%. He was advised to put Doron in a special school for the handicapped because with 20% vision in each eye, he was unable to see properly, and he would never be able to drive an automobile. They told my cousin that he had some developmental problem in which his vision had not developed to the normal level. A year later, I had an opportunity to travel to London and brought with me an ophthalmoscope. Armed with this instrument, I examined the exterior and interior of Doron's eye. During the examination, I discovered a peculiar reflex. In opthalmological terms, this is a certain indication or a sign that this child might have a condition known as Keratoconus. This is not an uncommon condition: I have many patients with similar problems. It is a condition in which the front of the eye actually begins to come to a point, instead of being rounded like a baseball. Therefore, the name Conus or Keratoconus, or pointed cornea. I immediately referred him to a skilled London ophthalmologist who was familiar with contact lenses and their usefulness in this condition. Much to the amazement and surprise of his parents (and to me, too), Doron was fitted with contact lenses and achieved 20/20 vision which he enjoys to this day.

I specifically chose this type of case as a basis for discussing

Keratoconus because it is such an important condition for so many people. Ophthalmologists who deal with contact lenses look for this condition and are familiar with it, but many eye doctors do miss it because they are not contact lens oriented. The actual cause of this condition is not known, but the following theories have been advanced:

1. It is a degeneration of the ccorneal tissue itself.
2. It is an aberration of growth; a developmental defect.
3. It has been associated with hypothyroidism (low thyroid).
4. It has occurred in cases of long illness.
5. It has occurred in cases of malnutrition.
6. To a certain extent, it is a hereditary disease.
7. The English feel it is caused by severe and intense itching and rubbing of the eyes.

No accurate figures are available, but it is generally believed that one person in eight thousand has this condition.

Some symptoms of this condition include the following:

1. Decreasing vision in one eye.
2. Development of nearsightedness and astigmatism.
3. Changing astigmatism.
4. Ghost images. A patient will state he sees a ghost above certain letters, a symptom almost diagnostic.
5. Munson's Sign. This is seen when a patient looks down and the cone indents the lower lid.

There are a number of ingenious ways to treat this condition:

1. There is a type of hard contact lens with a special design known as Sopercone Lenses. Joseph Soper of Houston designed this lens which has proved effective in many cases.
2. In the piggy back technique of Joseph Baldone, M.D., of New Orleans, a soft lens is placed on the cone and a hard lens is fitted over it. Thus a patient having cones in both eyes would wear four contact lenses. These patients wear them well and like them.
3. A new lens called a Saturn Lens has a hard center and a soft rim. In many cases this works quite well.
4. When the cone is so severe and so advanced that contact lenses will not work, there is an operation called Epikeratophakia. In this procedure, the top layer of the cornea is removed and a new cornea is sewn on to the patient's

own cornea to flatten his cone; afterward a contact lens can be satisfactorily fitted.

5. When all else fails, a cornea transplant often brings dramatic results. This involves removing the conical cornea completely and sewing on a new cornea.

Special Note: Report in *Archives of Ophthalmology, 1968*

Although contact lenses are the only means of correcting this condition outside of surgery, some professionals believe (as I do), this condition can develop in certain patients wearing contact lenses.

9

"I'M GETTING SO OLD, DOCTOR"

"I'm getting old, Dr. Jordanreid," Krim sighed. "And I just can't stand the idea of bifocals. I'd rather not wear glasses at all."

"That's foolish," the ophthalmologist replied. "It's dangerous for you to go without glasses. You're farsighted, and you don't see well up close, either. You're liable to have an accident if you drive, and besides, you'll have to give up reading completely if you don't wear some kind of glasses."

"Isn't there another way, doctor?"

"Yes, there is," replied Dr. Jordanreid. "I just wanted to test how motivated you are. there are several contact lens alternatives."

"What do you mean by alternatives?"

"There are a number of hard and soft bifocal contact lense currently on the market, but most practitioners agree that the concept of monovision, fitting one eye for distance and one for near, offers the greatest chance for success."

"Sounds like one vision."

"Well, not exactly. In this technique," Dr. Jordanreid explained, "we fit one contact lens to see far away and fit a second contact lens, on your other eye, for reading."

"Does that work? I thought we needed both eyes to see at distance and both eyes to read."

"Surprisingly enough," said Dr. Jordanreid, "approximately eighty to ninety percent of patients who are farsighted find that they do quite well using this principle of monovision. If it works for you, you won't need to wear bifocal flasses."

"That certainly would make me much happier," Krim smiled.

After a complete eye examination, Dr. Jordanreid proceeded

37

to select one contact lens for distance and place that in her right eye. Krim is right handed and an eye dominance test indicated she is right-eyed, too. He then placed a reading contact lens in her left eye and showed her that with her right lens she saw in the distance, and the left contact lens aided her 'near vision.' After all the necessary instructions relating to contact lenses, Krim left the office, no longer "feeling old."

10

GOOD NEWS/BAD NEWS

The buzz of conversation stopped when Dr. Arjay entered the small meeting room. "I'm very pleased you were all able to attend today," he began. "I feel it's important that potential contact lens patients are informed on the care and use of contact lenses before they're dispensed. This avoids many problems later. A recent communique from the Center for Disease Control in Atlanta confirms the findings of many ophthalmologists. Negligence in the proper care of contact lenses and symptoms that are ignore may result in the loss of an eye from parasitic infection." The ten men and women stirred uneasily in their chairs. "I don't mean to alarm you; rather, I'm here to caution you. Regular check-ups, meticulous care of your contact lenses and visits to your ophthalmologist when symptoms occur will help prevent this from happening to you."

"I wear a lot of make-up, Doctor. Are certain ones better than others?"

"Yes they are, Merle. Liquid eyeliner is preferred over pencil eyeliner because it doesn't run or flake and it's best to use soap that doesn't contain cold cream or deodorants. Soaps with these ingredients can leave a film on the fingertips that is easily trans-ferred to the lenses. This can result in smudging, irritation or interfere with proper wetting."

"Can we keep our nails polished?"

"No problem, Bev."

"Dr. Arjay, I blow dry my hair," Chuck volunteered and added sheepishly, "I sometimes use hair spray."

"Blow dryers don't present a problem, Chuck, but use hair

spray with caution. Spraying your hair before inserting your lenses is the safest way to go."

"I go to the beauty shop. Any danger from sitting under a dryer?"

"I'd avoid hot air dryers, Audrey. They tend to dry tears and lenses. A corneal abrasion could result from lack of lubrication. I would like to move on and discuss eye problems that restrict the use of contact lenses. If any of you has been diagnosed with chronic hyperemia of the conjunctiva, you might want to reconsider wearing contact lenses. This condition involves the mucuous membrane lining the inner surface of the eyelids and covering the front part of the eyeball. Patients with this condition will probably find contact lenses only add to the irritation of the eyes. Acute bacterial conjunctivitis holds a slightly rosier picture. Once the condition is treated and the infection cleared, it is possible for the patient to consider contact lenses."

"What about diabetes? I'm a borderline diabetic."

"Only uncontrolled diabetes is contraindicated."

You said this was a good news-bad news seminar, Doctor. How about some of the good stuff?"

"Right you are, Audrey. The good news is that people like you who come to learn and ask questions usually have a high success rate with contact lenses. Near sighted people do well, too. That should make you happy, Chuck."

"What about colored lenses? Can they really make my brown eyes blue?"

"They sure can…if you're a soft lens wearer."

"But are they safe?"

"They're safe, Bev, but as with any contact lenses, care must be taken. Care of your eyes and care of your lenses. I would also like to recommend that the ladies keep their nails clipped to avoid scratching their eyes or tearing their lenses."

"Are there tools or instruments that help insert or remove lenses?"

"Yes, Merle. As your ophthalmologist to show them to you after he determine the type lens you need."

"What if I find I don't like wearing contacts or discover they feel awkward or uncomfortable? Can I get a refund?"

"Each case is different, Audrey. It's wise to discuss this with your doctor at the time of your examination. That concludes our seminar. Each of you will receive instructions specific to your needs when your contact lenses are dispensed. Just remember…any discomfort, change in vision or irritation to your eyes needs prompt attention by your ophthalmologist."

11

CONTACT LENS HISTORY

Today, approximately, twenty to twenty-two million people are wearing contact lenses and, approximately four and a half million people are wearing contact lenses on an extended wear basis, that is they are leaving them in their eyes overnight or to varying periods of time. It is expected that by 1989 or 1990 the number of people wearing extended wear contact lenses alone will reach some ten million.

The history of contact lenses is a fascinating one and I thought my readers might enjoy some of the highlights in their development.

Dr. Thomas Young, on the basis of a paper written in 1798 and presented in 1801, is credited with conceiving the idea for contact lenses. He described an instrument, later called a hydrodiascope, with which he sought to abolish the optical disadvantages of the corneal curvature. He fitted a microscope lens on the end of a glass tube ¼inch long, filled the tube with water, and then applied this to his eye. The idea was to eliminate the corneal from the dioptric system of the eye and substitute for it a regularly ground lens. The following is a quotation from Young's paper: "From a small microscope destined for botanical research. I removed a biconvex lens of approximately 20 millimeters in focal length; I fixed it in a small tube 5 millimeters long, after having coated the tube with a little wax, and after having filled it three quarters with almost cold water, I applied it to my eye in such a way that the cornea half entered the tube, and was everywhere in contact with the water. The eye immediately became far sighted."

42

In 1827 Airy reported in the Transactions of the Cambridge Philosophical Society a remarkable observation that he had made concerning one of his own eyes. He thus made the first diagnosis of astigmatism and described the use of astigmatic lenses to correct this type of refraction. At about the same time Herschel proposed the use of contact lenses filled with a transparent gelatinous substance to be placed in contact with the cornea as a means of correcting regular and irregular astigmatism. To quote Herschel, "In some cases of malformation of the cornea, it would be interesting to examine if some transparent animal gel placed in contact with this coat and maintained by a glass capsule could not possibly render distinct the vision."

At about this time three scientists, working independently of each other, first attempted to adapt a contact lens to the human eye. These men were A.E. Fick of Zurich, E. Kalt of Paris, and August MullerGladbach of Kiel.

Fick's work appeared in the Klinische Monatsblatter fur Augenheilkunde in August, 1888. Fick called his contact lens "Kontackt Brille." It was a small cup of thin glass made up of a spherical segment with concentric and consequently parallel faces. The space between the lends and the eye was filled with a liquid of the same refraction index as that of the cornea. Fick first experimented with rabbits. After removing the eyelids, he filled the pocket with liquid plaster and made a series of plaster molding on the eyes of living rabbits. The moldings showed that the radious of curvature of a rabbit's cornea is almost equal that of the sclera; the rabbit's eye is almost a perfect sphere. Cups of blown glass were then shaped on these moldings. After a series of trials, Fick found that a lens of a well-chosen shape can adhere to the eyeball with no eyelid to hold it in place; it is solidly applied against the eyeball or adheres to it by atmospheric pressure. He also investigated a number of solutions to be used between the eye and the lens and finally tried sodium chloride solution to which he added compounds such as alcohol glycerin and eventually a 2% glucose solution.

After his experiments with rabbits, Fick studied eye moldings taken on human corpses; these showed that in man the corneal radius is shorter than the scleral radius. Fick first tried these lenses on himself and was able to tolerate them for 2 hours. In the summer of 1887 he contacted the director of the Zeiss Company and asked him to construct a contact lens according to the following dimensions: the base of the cup of the sphere for the cornea was to be 7mm in diameter; the radius of curvature of this cup was to measure 8mm; and the4 sclera was to be 3mm wide and have a radius of curvature of 12mm. The faces of the cornea were to be parallel to each other and cut and polished, and the free edge of the scleral part was to be carefully polished. The total lens weight was to be 0.5 grams. Of the first six patients whom Fick fitted with contact lenses, five had irregular astigmatism and one had keratoconus.

Kalt's work was presented at the March 20, 1888 session of the Academia de Medecine by a P. Panas, who apparently was in charge of the hospital department in which Kalt was chief resident. Panas reported that kalt had treated two patients at the Hotel Dieu who had keratoconus: "One of our patients who could hardly count fingers at 0.5 meters immediately saw his vision improve to the point of reading 26-millimeter type at a distance of 5 meters. At close range, he could read the newspaper. Optical correction is thus achieved in a very satisfactory manner. The future will tell us about the curative effect of such lenses."

In 1889 August Muller-Gladbach, who was about 25 years of age, published a thesis in which he developed a theory of contact lenses; he called them Hornhautlinsen. Because he was nearsighted about 14.00 D, he obtained the services of an optician in Berlin to make him a pair of contact lenses to his specifications. The radius of curvature of the posterior surface of the corneal part measured 8mm and the scleral radius measured 12mm. For his myopia, the anterior curvature had a radius of 10mm; thus he corrected his nearsightedness from -14.00 to -0.50 D. However, he could never wear the lenses for more than 30 minutes. He recognized that the cause of his intolerance was not the lens on the cornea but the crushing of the conjuctival vessels by the edge of the lens. He made several attempts to solve this difficulty, but he finally gave up.

In 1892 Sulzer reported fitting two patients with ground contact lenses, which were made by the Zeiss Company.

Heine, reporting to the Thirteenth International Congress of Ophthalmology held in Amsterdam of 1929, described a method of fitting contact lenses by means of a trial set, consisting of a large number of contact lenses that were made for him by the Zeiss Company.

Dallos, working at Professor Grosz's clinic in Budapest in 1932, perfected a personal molding technique, which improved on Csapody's method; he presented the details of this technique in 1933. He obtained the negative with Negacoll, a hydrophilic colloid that, then boiled in water, foams into a homogeneous mass. When cooled to body temperature, it solidfies in 30 to 60 seconds, depending on its water content. It preserves the most minute particularities of the surface that it reproduces, while remaining as elastic as rubber. Dallos subsequently moved to London and became a manufacturer of lenses, establishing centers in Utrecht and London. William Feinbloom was the first American to use plastic in the construction of contact lenses. He reported in 1937 on a lens having a glass corneal portion and a plastic scleral portion.

Theodore Obrig introduced an all-plastic scleral contact lens in 1940. This lens was completely transparent in both corneal and scleral portions. Obrig is also known for introducing the use of fluorescein in ultraviolet light for checking the fit of contact lenses.

Norman Bier of England introduced a minimum-clearance, fluidless, preformed contact lens because it includes a transitional curve between the corneal and scleral curves. This lens is fenestrated, having a perforation at the temporal limbus.

The wide-angle lens was introduced in 1946 by Nissel in England. Although it is also a ventilated, minimum-clearance lens, it differs from the transcurve lens in that there is a flat transition between the corneal and scleral portions of the lens; it serves the same purpose as the transition curve in the transcurve lens, however, to allow limbal clearance.

This lens was introduced into the United States in 1950 and was known as the Mueller-Welt fluidless contact lens. The lens is fitted in such a manner that there is a layer of tears between the lens and the cornea and a cushion of air in the layer of tears between the lens and the cornea and a cushion of air in the form of one or more air pockets under the scleral portion of the lens. It actually was first invented as a glass lens by Mueller-Welt in

1925. I started fitting this lens in 1951, shortly after its introduction.

The first corneal plastic contact lens was introduced in 1948, and credit for it is given to Kevin M. Tuohy, a technician who originally worked in Theodore Obrig's laboratory. This first lens was approximately 11mm in diameter and 0.4mm thick, it was fitted flatter than the optic cap of the cornea.

The micorlens, approximately 9.5mm in diameter, 0.2mm thick with a single curve, and fitted 3.00 to 4.00 D flatter than the optic cap of the cornea, was introduced in 1951 simultaneously by three persons; Wilhelm Soehnges of Germany, Frank Dickinson of England, and John Neill of America.

The contous principle of fitting which is embodied in a corneal lens having multiple inside radii, was introduced by Norman Bier in 1955.

Corneal lenses currently being constructed are small and thin; they are either parallel to the cornea or they vault the apex of the cornea, in which case they are called apical clearance lenses. They are now fitted as small as 5 to 7mm in diameter, and I have even heard reports of lenses 4mm in diameter being fitted experimentally. Most recent advancement include lenses made of hydrophilic and oxygen permeable materials; these are known as "soft" lens and liquid gas permeable lenses.

Many names have been given to the hydrophilic lenses, among which are the following:
1. Gel contact lenses.
2. Gel-kontakt flexible lenses.
3. Hydrogel contact lenses.
4. Hydragel contact lenses.
5. Soflenses.
6. Gelatin contact lenses.

Hydrophilic contact lenses were first developed by Professor Otto Wichterle of the institute of Macromolecular Chemistry in Prague, Czechoslovakia. They are made of hydrogel polydioxyethylene methacrylate, which is hydrophilic. Fifty to sixty percent of the lens weight is water when it is fully saturated; it can be compressed and thus water can be removed from it as one would squeeze moisture from a sponge. The lenses have to be kept in an aqueous solution (a solution of 0.5% sodium bicarbonate in distilled water is recommended). When hydrated, the lenses can easily be bent but will return to their original shape when released. When dry, they become flat and brittle and must be soaked for several hours before they are inserted into the eye. They are produced in two basic diamters-10 and 13mm. The back surface is parabolic, the central portion being 7.2mm in radius, plus or minus 0.3mm. The thickness of these lenses is greater than that of standar corneal lenses—a—10.00 D lens may be 1mm thick; a—1.00 D lens may be 0.3mm thick.

Some problems that have been encountered so far by wearers and dispensers of these lenses are the following:

1. Visual acuity is not as great as with methylmethacrylate lenses.
2. Because the lens follows the corneal shape, in corneal astigmatism that is over 2.00 D an asitmatic front furface is produced. To overcome this, the central portion of the lens can be produced in a hard plastic to a diameter of 1 to 2mm.
3. Fluorescein cannot be used to evaluate the fit since the lens absorbs the stain.

The Soflens, manufactured by Bausch & Lomb, was the first of the hydrophilic contact lenses to gain FDA approval in the United States.

In 1965 the first licensing agreement between a United States company and a Soviet block government was made. The national Patent corporation of New York and Polytechna, the official Czechoslovakian licensing agency, arranged a licensing agreement by which the national Patent Corporation was to handle the Wichterle lens in the Western Hemisphere. It was also allowed sublicensing rights in the original agreement. These sublicensing rights were exercised in the case of two contact lens manufacturers, neither of whom ever marketed the hydrophilic lens on a national basis. In October of 1966, Bausch & Lomb announed that it had entered into a patent sublicense agreement with the National Patent Corporation that granted Bausch & Lomb an exclusive right to manufacture and sell hydrophilic lenses under certain United States and other patents. The patents are those of Wichterle and others. Hydrophilic lenses or hydrogels, like most plastics, are made up of giant molecules. In the case of polymethylmethacrylate, which is universally used in contact lens construction, the methylmethacrylate monomer is treated with a catalyst such as benzoyl peroxide, causing the molecules to join together in long strands. Thus the methylmethacrylate monomer becomes polymethylmethacrilate, a polymer; this interaction causes the monomer, which is a liquid, to change to a solid as it polymerizes.

Polymers, as a general rule, are hydrophobic or water hating, polymethylmethacrylate being a prime example of this hydrophobic tendency. The reason for the hydrophobic nature of this molecule is that chemically it has little or no free oxygen or OH (hydroxyl) groups to which tears or water can become attached. Though not as common, there are also polymers that are so hydrophilic that they actually swell and take up water much like a sponge. Polyvinyl alcohol and methylcellulose are examples of such polymers both of which should be recognizable to contact lens practitioners as they are commonly used in wetting solutions. Each of these polmer molecules has an abundance of OH ions, which accounts for its wetting potential. The chemical make up of the hydrogel lens is polydioxyethylene methacrylate. The presence of three oxygen atoms plus an OH group in each molecular unit makes the polymer hydrophilic instead of hydrophobic. Otherwise it has essentially the same formula as polymethylmethacrylate. Bausch & Lomb has stated that the material that it uses in construction of its gel lens is a polymer of hydroxyethylmethacrylate cross lengths with ethylene glycol dimethacrylate. This is probably essentially the same material as introduce by Wichterle in 1964. Hydrophilic lenses are therefore made from a solid colloidal material that consists of particles, a continuous dispersion medium, and a stabilizing agent. If a liquid colloid (a sol) is to be changed to a solid colloid (a gel), the liquid must be immobilized. The resultant plastic is polydioxyethylene methacrylate. Aside from the presence of three oxygen atoms and one OH group in each molecular unit, its formula is the same as that of polymethylmethacrylate. This important chemical difference makes a cross-length polymer hydrophilic, resulting in dehydrated and hydrated states.